THANK YOU TO OUR PARTNERS!

PickNIC is a shared vision. As the project leader, I want to personally thank the individuals and organizations who have sponsored PickNIC 2014! Each is investing in America's youth – our future.

— Ingrid Kohlstadt MD, MPH

Phil Meldrum; President, FoodMatch; Board Member of OldWays

Joan Adeloye; President, Best Way Snacks, Inc.

Jean-François Larivière; Bee Healthy Farms, LLC

Pete Vas Dias; Nature's Stance, makers of Xylichew Gum

Pete Truby; Salazon Chocolate Co.

Eric Eddings; CEO, Sahale Snacks

Norman Kauffman; Kauffman's Fruit Farm and Market

Steve Baker; Flavrz Organic Beverages, LLC

Raymond Chung; President, Cruncha Ma-Me Edamame Snacks

Willow King and Mara King; Co-CEOs, Ozuké

Robert Freeland; CEO, Go Raw, Inc.

Annegret Berndt

Blaker and Blaker Chiropractic

David Bley; President, Bley Advertising

Jonathan Collin, MD; Publisher, Townsend Letter

Russell M. Hostetler, MD

Davinder S. Khanna; President, Accounting Heritage Group, LLC

Sanjaya N. Joshi and Susan D. Baird-Joshi

Elisabeth "Mutti" Kohlstadt and Horst Kohlstadt

Kathryn Poleson, DMD and Thomas Dowdy, DDS

Peter Poon

Stephany Porter, ND; Director, The Bodhi Clinic

Ellis Richman; NutriBee National Nutrition Competition, Inc.

Jacob Teitelbaum, MD; author of *From Fatigued to Fantastic*

David and Mattie Tenzer

Alan Weiss, MD and Kim Weiss, RN; Annapolis Integrative Medicine

2014 EDITION

PickNIC™

PICK NUTRITIOUS INGREDIENTS COST-EFFECTIVELY

2014 EDITION

PickNIC™

PICK NUTRITIOUS INGREDIENTS COST-EFFECTIVELY

100 BEST BROWN BAG LUNCHES

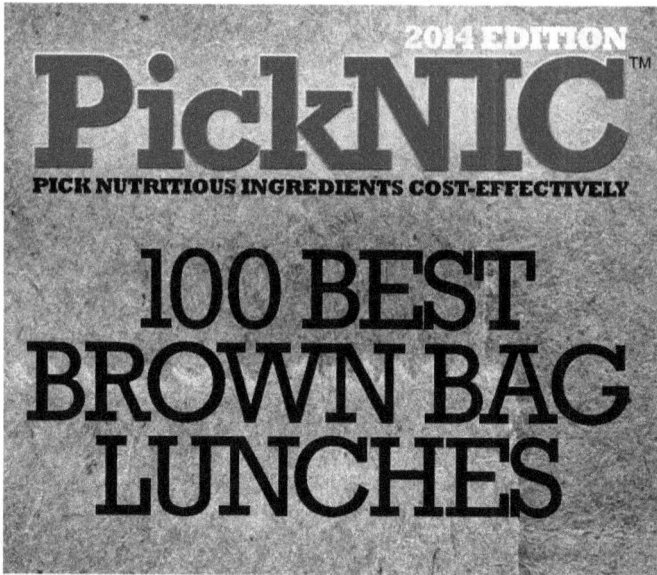

by **Ingrid Kohlstadt, MD, MPH**
Fellow of the American College of Nutrition
Fellow of the American College of Preventive Medicine
Faculty Associate, Johns Hopkins Bloomberg School of Public Health
Editor, Advancing Medicine with Food and Nutrients, 2nd Edition, 2013
Founding Director of NutriBee National Nutrition Competition, Inc.

Contents

Preface

Simplifying nutritious

The ember that sparked PickNIC was a rapid succession of requests I received in 2013 from kids, parents, grandparents and doctors. Each request had simplicity at its core.

Youth participating in a nutrition engagement program wanted nutritious foods that appealed to them. They also wanted to be more involved in family food preparation.

Parents were asking for simpler solutions which took less time and less money. Grandparents sought to help improve children's health, and they wanted to do so in ways that would be viewed as supportive.

Several doctors in primary care and preventive medicine and two Johns Hopkins medical students initially voiced their request for practical tools to guide their patients' food selection. One benefit of crowd-source funding this public health initiative is that it provided us additional texture on PickNIC's anticipated users. Health care professionals of many specialties are among our backers and supporters.

Exploring the components of best

PickNIC stands for Pick Nutritious Ingredients Cost-effectively. It was developed as a public health initiative to simplify and energize the brown bag lunch. Since brown bag lunches are generally served cold and forego refrigeration for a few hours, taste at room temperature and food safety were emphasized.

There's no one store where all of the PickNIC foods could be found. The PickNIC team sought ethnically diverse cuisine and journeyed off-the-beaten-health-trail.

Foods needed to taste good to most taste-testers. The voices and savory sentiments of taste testers were highly considered, especially the opinions of the youth. Then, each entry has been vetted by a leading authority on nutrition and food safety.

Reaching 100

We selected 80 foods suitable as an entrée for a brown bag lunch. Forty are home packed and need overnight refrigeration. Forty do not need overnight refrigeration which allows them to be mailed as care packages or placed in lockers. Also, ten entrées are snack bars. The food technology advances have diversified the selection of healthful snack bars. Our list includes 10 beverages and 10 desserts.

Using this resource

PickNIC is a resource for new ideas, practical tips, and cost and time saving solutions. It is not a metric for the best foods for any one individual. Remember that foods that are not listed in PickNIC may be very nutritious. PickNIC selected among nutritious foods for taste, appeal, practicality and cost, not only nutritional value.

The 2014 edition is the inaugural PickNIC. The PickNIC team welcomes suggestions for future editions.

100 Bests in Brown Bag Lunches

40 Bests in home-packed brown bag lunches

1. The pizza party revamp!

Health-aware kids no longer need to miss out on the school pizza party. We like Go Raw's Pizza Flax Snax. These sprouted grain and tomato crackers awaken the same taste buds as pizza. Yet they are healthful and digestible!

PickNIC agrees with the package claim, "All content has been dried under 105°F and all seeds have been sprouted, releasing enzymes which make them healthier and easier to digest. Sprouted seeds are among the most nutritionally dense foods on the planet."

Add a few side toppings such as grated cheddar cheese, fresh basil or cilantro, or Divina olives.

2. Dolmas

Mediterranean rice-filled grape leaves are an American favorite food waiting to be discovered. When I invite youth to try what may be their first dolma, I strive to have them coming back for more. Dolmas taste best, are most popular and better digested when the grape leaves are soft and the rice stuffing is firm. Divina is the brand with which I debut dolmas to America's youth.

While taste is initially why Divina caught PickNIC's attention, we then became impressed with Divina's dedication to cultural authenticity, food safety and customer service. Divina dolmas can be ordered online, purchased in brick and mortar stores and selected from the antipasto bar at Whole Foods.

3. Cabbage a la the globe

Cabbage is the world's traditional food. Whether it's called kimchee, sauerkraut or kohl, pickled cabbage is packed with health benefits. After a long search I found the authenticity and taste appeal needed to showcase cabbage in youth nutrition programs. I called the company owners, excited that I had finally found a partner for rediscovering cabbage, Ozuké.

PickNIC agrees with Ozuké's tag line, "The best pickled things." PickNIC enjoyed ruby calendula kraut, citrus & ginger kraut, and kimchi with anchovy and pear. These and other pickled vegetables can be purchased at ozuke.com.

Ozuké products are labeled "keep refrigerated." Of the products that require refrigeration only after opening, consider Andre Laurent coastal style ready to serve sauerkraut.

4. Egg-celence explained

Give hardboiled eggs the best chance possible. A kitchen egg slicer and egg timer help engage kids in the kitchen, and add to the joy of eating eggs. Salt, pepper or mustard packets accompanying a hardboiled egg can add to appeal.

Not only are eggs naturally packaged, hard-boiled eggs are better for you than eggs that are scrambled, fried, poached or baked. Hard-boiling allows the delicate good-for-you neurolipids to cook before exposure to air. Air oxidizes egg nutrients and damages them.

Invest the extra $ for free-range, organic eggs. PickNIC extends a special thanks to Dr. Kathryn Poleson, whose lovely photography confers organic hens' eggs with the innate beauty of a floral bouquet.

Consider decorating hard-boiled eggs with a simple-to-use, natural dye:

Step 1. Pour frozen blueberries into a large bowl.

Step 2. Fully cover hard-boiled eggs in the bowl of frozen berries.

Step 3. Place the bowl of eggs and berries in the refrigerator, allowing the berries to slowly thaw. This usually takes 4-6 hours.

Step 4. Remove the eggs from the bowl and place them on a paper towel to dry. Enjoy the eggs bedecked with purple polka dots.

5. Banana + cashew or almond butter

This electrolyte powerhouse fruit is best eaten with dietary fat. Consider enjoying a banana with cashew or almond butter.

The nut butter can be spread directly onto the banana one slice at a time. Use firm bananas and soft nut butter. The challenge with nut butter is that if it's natural and not processed, it tends to get hard over time. That is especially true of colder, drier climates. Freshly ground nut butter is often sold at country markets and high-end grocers. Warming a glass jar of nut butter and then stirring it can help soften nut butter that became hard over time.

6. Yogurt: Yes, but which kind?

Does your brand meet the following criteria:

- No artificial sweeteners
- Minimal sugar
- Live active cultures
- Yogurt made from goat or sheep milk is preferred, because of fewer naturally occurring hormones than yogurt made from cow milk. This was not one

of our criteria but is important to note on an individual basis when certain medical conditions are present.

There's one more note of caution. Yogurts high in protein may be more difficult to digest. The protein is the component of milk associated with allergies.

Brands PickNIC has enjoyed are Pequea Valley, Maple Hill Creamery, Old Chatham Sheepherding Company, Liberté (goat yogurt line), and Redwood Hill Farm. Siggi's yogurt tubes are new and popular.

For a non-dairy yogurt consider So Delicious brand. Choose the unsweetened cultured coconut milk or plain cultured almond milk.

7. Lettuce-wrapped veggie burger

Choose your favorite veggie burger. Serve it as a lettuce wrap garnished with a freshly sliced tomato or carefully chosen (avoid sugar) barbeque sauce or salsa.

8. Veggie pancakes

Consider vegetable pancakes which can be stored frozen. They can be pan grilled without thawing and served warm or cold. Dr. Praeger's offers broccoli, spinach, zucchini and carrot, corn and root vegetable pancakes. The sweet potato pancakes are a favorite any time of year, especially during Hanukkah when served as latkes. PickNIC has a favorite pancake topping, Kauffman's no-sugar-added fruit butters. Choose among apple spice,

pumpkin, pear and peach when purchasing online from Kauffmansfruitfarm.com or from your local Amish Market. The fruit butter gift boxes are easily shipped, making it possible to help pack students' lunches from a distance.

9. Celery stuffed with raisins and sesame or almond butter

Sometimes called ants on a log, this kids' lunch classic is worth a second look. Celery becomes easier to digest with a dietary fat, and the raisins add the right amount of sweetness for a child's palate. Seed butter such as sesame and sunflower creates a nut-free version of ants on a log.

10. Hummus and a rice cake

This is a favorite variation of rice and beans, that's portable. Single packets of hummus are convenient.

Dip and rise are not opposites when it comes to hummus. The National Football League made hummus the official dip of the NFL. Both enjoyed a rise in popularity.

11. Tempeh sauté

Tempeh can be purchased refrigerated. Prepare it by slicing quarter-inch strips. Prepare an iron or stainless steel skillet on low heat and stir-fry the strips with sesame oil and soy sauce. Add fresh basil, fresh cilantro, Italian seasoning or broccoli raab. Tempeh can be served warm or cold.

Tempeh is available with flax seeds. Coconut curry tempeh is a tasty variation.

12. Crudité (raw veggies) rediscovered

There's one good thing I know about most party vegetable platters. There is usually some left for the last person in the reception line, even at nutrition programs.

Give crudité another chance. Here are 3 simple changes to move crudité to the top of the charts:

- Choose mandolin-sliced vegetables. The diagonal slices have eye appeal, taste better and are better for you, because they are more easily digested.

- Select cucumber, green bean, romaine lettuce heart, thinly coined carrots, jicama sticks, and thinly sliced radishes.

- Add a new dipping sauce. We like tahini, pesto, tamarind chutney (salsa), salad dressings by Tessemae's and the Arugula (salad rocket) Salsa recipe on Taste.com.au. Jake & Amos salsas can be purchased through Kauffmansfruitfarm.com .

13. Cucumber with dairy or a dairy alternative

Cucumber slices with cream cheese lends itself to lunch. For those who need to avoid dairy products, consider Go Veggie cream cheese alternative.

The cucumber dairy combination has global appeal. For a Greek lunch pack tzatziki. For Turkish flare choose cacik. Add Indian spices and call it raita.

14. Muesli

Swiss efficiency extends to oatmeal. Swiss muesli is oats and dried fruit mixed with fermented dairy. The mixture self-prepares in 6 hours. The health benefits are impressively corroborated by the latest scientific research on the microbiome.

Here I share my own family's muesli recipe. We call it Mutti's Muesli.

Ingredients:

2 cups	Rolled oats
1 cup	Yogurt or Kefir

1 cup	Nut milk (almond, hazelnut, coconut)
½ cup	Fruit juice (cherry, prune, orange)
1 Tablespoon	Lemon juice
1 Teaspoon	Cinnamon
Optional grain:	Ground flaxseed, teff, quinoa or pecans
Optional fruit:	Berries, bananas, or apricots (fresh or dried)

Preparation:

Combine and mix 6-12 hours beforehand and refrigerate.

15. Olives

A small jar or reusable plastic container featuring olives is an enjoyable side dish. PickNIC asked Phil Meldrum of Food Match to advise us on how to introduce olives to youth. He recommends starting with castelvetrano olives, pitted kalamata olives, and olive bruschetta. Ever since, we've experienced a surge in olive sampling.

16. Beet + goat cheese + basil salad

Slice some pickled beets, crumble in some goat cheese and pluck a few basil leaves from your potted garden if available (an herb shaker works) and you have a fast and tasty salad.

17. Trail mix

Designate a reusable bag or small metal lunch box as the snack box. Consider using it daily and filling it weekly with raisins, dried apricots and favorites from the PickNIC list.

18. Fresh pomegranate and watermelon

It doesn't take more than a few sliced pomegranates or watermelons to turn a kitchen into a staged crime scene. Forego the mess but not the message these healthful foods send to the body.

Here are some ideas for the persistent. Pomegranate seeds are sold in small containers, already processed. They refrigerate well for up to a week. Pomegranate juice can be removed from clothing and kitchen cloths with hot water, no soap. Watermelon can be put into the blender and poured into small leak-proof freezer containers, and added to lunches over a period of time.

19. Fresh papaya and pineapple

This is a lunchtime favorite of Dr. Jacob Teitelbaum. The enzymes in these fruits are a calorie-free energy boost.

20. Grilled corn-on-the-cob

Corn may have originated in the New World, but grilled corn-on-the-cob is popular around the world and is served warm or cold.

21. Oven-roasted Brussels sprouts, broccoli or cauliflower

Because cruciferous vegetables are especially important for helping the body remove toxic chemicals, it's worth trying a variety and preparing them in different ways. Roasting cruciferous vegetables makes them more easily digested.

22. Pumpkin butter

Pumpkin, pear and apple butter without added sugar are delicious old ways. The word "butter" formerly described any spread or sauce. Combine no-sugar-added pumpkin butter with fresh cheese or quark. Fruit butters can be found at local Amish markets and online at KauffmansFruitFarm.com.

23. Edamame

For centuries the Japanese have cultivated soybeans for a soft, thin pod and large, sweet seeds. These exceptional soybeans are called edamame, and are cultivated specifically for human consumption.

Edamame can be purchased fresh or frozen and then steamed in the pod. They are lightly salted and served as an appetizer, warm or cold. The seeds are squeezed out of the pod at the table and the pods are discarded.

24. Soft ripened cheese

Soft cheeses such as brie and camembert are among the most digestible dairy products. Instead of eating cheese with bread, consider toasted nori (a variety of seaweed) or freshly sliced fruit.

Important food safety message: Purchase a small wheel rather than a slice, because the rind of the cheese protects it against unwanted bacteria. Always check the "Best by" date and keep refrigerated. Anyone who has been cautioned about *Listeria* should avoid eating soft ripened cheese.

25. Lox + fresh herbs on olive-oil sprayed cracker

Consider smoked salmon on bread and garnished with herbs. Most youth who sample salmon enjoy it.

Cost can be a barrier, so PickNIC researched this. In the mid-Atlantic area, packaged wild-caught sock-eye salmon sells for $1.50 per ounce.

Another practical barrier is minimizing dietary fat intake, since fish is a source of dietary fat. PickNIC suggests spraying extra virgin olive oil on a cracker and fresh herbs. A convenient spray bottled is marketed as Misto.

26. Borscht served with polenta

Red beets served Russian-style with cornbread served Italian-style is a fusion worth trying.

27. Gazpacho and tomato soup

The soups listed in 27 and 28 can be served warm or cold, making them a lunchtime favorite.

28. Butternut squash soup and carrot ginger soup

29. Tofurky beef brats with BBQ sauce

Tofu prepared as beef brats can be sliced and enjoyed with barbeque sauce. Since ketchup and barbeque sauce are a source of hidden sugar, we suggest label-reading.

30. Coconut bacon garnished potato salad

Add spicy flavor instead of fat or sugar. PickNIC likes Phoney Baloney's coconut bacon.

31. Mint chutney veggie sandwich

Make a sandwich with grilled vegetables. Add a slice of oven-baked turkey. Mint chutney is a flavorful spread.

32. Buy a bento box

Bento boxes are a longstanding Japanese lunch tradition. Most bento boxes PickNIC found contained a healthful assortment.

33. Tamales

Tamales can be eaten hot or cold and are eaten far beyond their village origins. Case in point, tamales can be purchased from Williams-Sonoma.

34. Antipasto

A side dish can be made from refrigerated jars of roasted sweet peppers, mozzarella cheese, sundried tomatoes and pearl onions.

Some grocery stores now feature antipasto bars. Consider filling several small containers, each ready to go for 1 day's lunch. The pickling process enhances food safety.

35. Grilled eggplant

PickNIC's favorite eggplant lunch preparation is the Middle Eastern tradition, baba ganoush.

36. Guacamole

Some people have mistakenly avoidedavocados because they are high in fat. A new look at this nutritional powerhouse fruit has shown that eating half of an avocado promotes satiety. In other words, even though avocados are high in calories compared to other fruits, they don't cause people to overeat.

37. Plum slices with ricotta cheese

Fresh plums can be halved and garnished with a spoonful of ricotta cheese.

38. Quinoa salad by Dr. Stephany Porter

For those who have time to prepare a lunch from scratch, this recipe is well-worth the invested effort.

Ingredients:

1 cup	quinoa
1 1/2 cups	cold water
1/4 tsp.	salt (optional)
1 cup	snow peas, shell peas, celery, or green beans
1 - 2	small carrots, peeled and sliced thin
1	medium cucumber, peeled and diced
1/4 cup	chopped fresh parsley, cilantro, or basil
1/2 cup	chopped walnuts, toasted sunflower seeds or toasted cashews

Dressing (optional):

2 Tbsp.	freshly squeezed lemon juice

1/4 cup	extra virgin olive oil
Pinch	cayenne, garlic powder or dried ginger

Preparation:

1. Rinse the quinoa 3 times and then cook it. Instructions vary with cooking method. When using a rice cooker, add 2 cups of cold water for each cup of quinoa and an optional ¼ teaspoon of salt.
2. Steam the carrots and green vegetables for 5 minutes or until tender-crisp. Drain. Rinse in cold water, and drain again.
3. Chop the tomatoes, herb and cucumber.
4. Combine veggies, walnuts, quinoa and the dressing in a large bowl.
5. Cover and chill.

39. California rolls

Vegetable sushi rolls are an excellent way to debut sushi. The sushi rolls which do not contain uncooked fish are generally food safe for a brown bag lunch.

40. Take the dare from down under: Vegemite-glazed pear slices

Vegemite, marmite, fish sauce, miso and other fermented dipping sauces have regional appeal. People generally like the fermented food from only their region. So far, there is no robust scientific explanation for this phenomenon. However, ongoing research on the human microbiome will probably reveal some surprising answers to this social and cultural phenomenon. The products can add dietary salt, but are otherwise probably beneficial. The benefits may be worth taking a cultural dare.

10 Snack bars that raise the bar

Congratulations go to the food manufacturers with tasty, healthful bars. Here we list snacks which have indeed raised the bar.

IMPORTANT: A snack bar is NEVER a complete snack. It is always designed to be consumed with a glass of water.

1. Birthday party bars

It's rare a health-aware family can enjoy the cake at a child's party. One way some families have navigated this unfortunate societal challenge is to reach for the bar. Invite the child to choose a snack bar to enjoy when the cake is being served. Being able to select a snack bar adds to the sense of empowerment and feeling included at the party.

We keep a variety of healthful, delicious bars wrapped with eye appeal aplenty. PickNIC favorites include GoMacro's Sunny Uplift (cherries and berries) and Thunderbird Energetica's Sweet Lemon Rain Dance.

2. Go Raw 100% Organic Spirulina Energy Bar

The seeds in this bar will sprout! The technology behind the achievement is impressive. Bringing live seeds into a snack bar involves the latest advances in food safety. Steps include the careful selection of non-GMO organic seeds, use of an optical sorter which removes seeds with imperfections, dehydrating the seeds at low temperatures and germinating the seeds in reverse osmosis treated water.

Spirulina adds a complex and interesting taste and nutrition from a different kingdom. While scientists debate Spirulina's nomenclature, all agree that it is neither plant nor animal and therefore has a unique set of nutrients and human health benefits.

3. Turkey (almond + cranberry) Epic Bar

Minimally processed lean meat served as a snack bar is a technical achievement. Epic Bar has truly raised the standard not only for snack bars but for poultry preparation. At first glance these bars may seem expensive. But when they are appropriately compared to a Thanksgiving meal, they are indeed a bargain.

Please note that each bar has a packet enclosed to keep it fresh. If you are dividing the bar in half for children's portions, be careful not to slice the packet.

4. Tanka Bison Bites

Those looking for a minimally processed bison bar should try Tanka. The bites are smaller than the bars and we preferred 1-3 of these as a lunch snack over the bar of bison.

5. Matt's Munchies Premium Fruit Snack

This is another snack that raises the bar. It's pureed fruit. That may sound straight-forward but it's not. Ambient temperature is an industrial challenge for fruit bars. When the weather turns cold, most fruit bars turn to rock. Leave them in your car for a few summer hours and you might lose half of the bar to the wrapper. By rolling this bar-shaped snack into a fruit roll-up, the wrapping paper help the fruit's consistency, naturally.

There's an additional benefit to the paper wrap. It can't be gobbled and gulped. The bar is portioned into appropriate bit-sized pieces, inviting consumers to slow down and enjoy the flavor.

These snacks have ample flavor. Our favorites are Choco-nana and mango.

6. Lamb (currant + mint) Epic Bar

This bar provides high quality animal protein which has been minimally processed. PickNIC thought the company's processing reflects careful attention to food safety.

7. Gluten-free oat bars

"Gluten–free" is not technically easy to achieve. When gluten-free is a dietary requirement Frankly Natural Bakers offers a tasty variety as does Bobo's Oat Bars. Thunderbird Energetica and Go Raw have gluten-free bars with diverse grains. Consider Go Raw's Banana Flax Seed bar.

8. Cocommune Bar

Vitamin companies are among the purveyors of snack bars. Few impressed us with cost-effectiveness and youth appeal. Overall we thought the Cocommune Bar by Designs for Health is worth a look.

9. Organic Active Greens Bar

PickNIC chose Organic Food Bar, Inc. as the best all round for taste, price and availability. We have sampled this bar widely among youth and it consistently receives thumbs-up reviews.

The price is favorable because most vendors will provide a case discount. One bar is two children's portions.

Please note that this recommendation may soon change. During our due diligence for PickNIC a document was located indicating that this snack bar has measurably high lead levels. The company has not responded to our request. We will look into this matter further.

10. Core by ProBar for those specifically looking for protein bars

Achieve the most plant protein 20 grams in 1 bar and gluten free, too. While this raises the bar on quality protein most people- child or adult – should make this 2 to 4 servings. The bar should be consumed with no less than 20 ounces of water. If someone has selected this bar because of gluten allergy they should be especially careful because when someone has an allergy to one protein they may easily acquire allergies to other proteins included in a high protein bar.

30 Best care package lunches

1. Freeze-dried pineapple

Freeze-drying preserves some of the pineapple's vitamins and enzymes. Even better, freeze-dried pineapple has the crunch of chips. We have 3 favorites: Funky Monkey's Java Lime, Simply Natural's freeze-dried pineapple and Danielle's tangy pineapple chips.

2. Fresh citrus

Kumquats are especially nutritious because the rinds and seeds can be eaten. As you rinse kumquats add a tablespoon of baking soda to the wash water.

3. Fresh kiwi fruit

Fresh kiwi fruit can be enjoyed in several ways. PickNIC has found it fun to include a kiwi spoon-knife. The spoon and knife combination makes it easy to cut the kiwi fruit in half and then scoop the fruit.

4. Applesauce and apple butter

When fresh apples aren't available we have two apple favorites: No-added-sugar apple butter by Kauffman's and organic applesauce with cinnamon single serving cups by various brands including Santa Cruz and 365. Kauffman's no-added-sugar products can be found at Kauffmansfruitfarm.com.

5. Dried plums

You pay less for prunes than for dried plums. People like dried plums better than prunes. Remember, the only difference is the name!

6. Freeze-dried cherries and berries

We like the Just Tomatoes Etc. brand. Try Just Cherries and Just Strawberries.

7. Carrot chips

Our favorite is Danielle's Spicy Carrot Chips.

8. Cereal or granola

Gluten-free granola or Nature's Path organic Mesa Sunrise (with raisins) cereal can be accompanied by a box of unsweetened rice milk for a brown-bag brunch. We suggest including a portable fruit such as a banana or freeze-dried berries.

9. Nori

Korean-style sesame toasted seaweed is available in single serving packets. We also like Feng Shui brand maki rolls, which combine seaweed with rice in a portable way.

10. Baked kale and baked beet chips

A few different brands are available. We liked them all. However, it's quite a savings to bake your own.

11. Plantain chips

Plantains are popular throughout the tropics. The advantage of purchasing dried plantains is that they were probably picked when fully ripened. The natural sweetness is greater than the fresh plantains picked green to be shipped north.

We liked plantain chips at a local African grocer. Plantain chips may be ordered from Best Way Snacks (bestwaysnacks.com) by calling 202-280-3770.

12. Marcona almonds

Nuts eaten 5 times per week have a health-extending effect comparable to fruits and vegetables. PickNIC saw this important research finding as a solid reason to introduce youth to a wide variety of nuts. The less common Marcona almonds have more taste appeal than other almonds, and may be worth an extra try.

13. Roasted pine nuts

Pine nuts have become more expensive due to drought conditions. However, for those wanting new nut flavors, this is one to try.

14. Peanuts and pistachio nuts in shell

A countertop bowl of nuts to shell is an expeditious way to reach 5 servings of nuts per week.

15. Roasted pumpkin seeds (popular around the world)

In African food stores you can find seeds from large pumpkins that have been peeled. These are called melon seeds or egusi. PickNIC thought these were the most affordable, healthful and delicious of the world's varieties. They are second only to the roasted seeds of our annual jack-o-lantern.

16. *Sacha inchi* snacks

In 1990 I participated in a Peruvian research project to develop the nutritional content of an indigenous plant called *Sacha inchi*, also known as the Incan peanut. The research was halted due to violence in the region and I subsequently heard little about this nutrient powerhouse.

Recently I found my long-lost favorite, gourmet style. *Sacha inchi* is now called savi seed and is sold in single serving packets by Vega brand. The cocoa-kissed savi seeds are especially tasty.

This snack is pricy but when the novelty is important or when there is a dietary restriction to nuts, consider savi seeds. Note that even though the translation suggests *Sacha inchi* is a nut, it is appropriately considered a seed.

17. Reclaiming popcorn

PickNIC set out to reclaim the delicious aroma and crunchy taste of freshly made popcorn. This was an ambitious endeavor since most popcorn is ruined with processed fats and excessive salt. However, we found one healthful, popcorn with tremendous crowd appeal. It's popcorn that pops right off the cob. The brand is Farmer's and it is readily available online.

One downside is that popcorn on the cob does require use of a microwave. We tried to pop it at a campfire and pan pop it, but these were technically unsuccessful. Even so, the novelty of popping corn off the cob renewed enthusiasm for nutritious popcorn among kids of all ages.

18. Wild salmon

After researching how smoked salmon could be portable for lunch, we came across Seabear brand. They offer single servings of wild salmon, and these 3.5 ounce packages do not require refrigeration before opening.

19. Cruncha Ma-Me

Edible soybeans (edamame) contain nutrients which support bone health and are regarded as a source of quality, plant-based protein. Cruncha Ma-Me is a non-GMO project verified, minimally processed edamame snack that has been freeze-dried to preserve essential nutrients. Cruncha Ma-Me uses all-natural seasonings, is gluten-free and Kosher certified. We are fans. The true-to-its-name crunch provides a welcome resemblance to chips and the spice blends make each flavor excitingly different. Visit Crunchamame.com for the rapidly expanding product list.

20. Indian snack mixes

Try khatta meetha, chiwdas and roasted fennel seeds. These snacks can be ordered on Amazon from various vendors or from the website of an Indian-based company named Haldiram. Saffron Road makes Bombay spice crunchy chick peas which are distributed by U.S. based American Halal Company.

21. Lentil and chia seed chips – old and new together

Lentil crackers are an Indian tradition called papads or papadum. Various U.S. companies now make lentil chips but the traditional Indian papads remain a favorite.

For a new style of multigrain chips consider Live Love Snack's chia and quinoa chips. We like the kale & sea salt flavor.

22. Potato chips

Lays baked potato chips is a readily available alternative
to fried potato chips. Our favorite is Popchips brand,
which is neither baked nor fried but popped.

23. Cashews and pecans

The cashew and pecan nut blends by Sahale Snacks are
exceptional at placing world-class gourmet flavors into a
bag. I now ask people lacking a palate for nuts to rethink
their opinion after trying Sahale Snack nut blends. Sing
Buri cashews showcases Thai cuisine and is seasoned
mostly with spices. Valdosta pecans are a culinary
tribute to American southern traditions. These can be
purchased at Sahalesnacks.com and at Costco stores
nationwide.

For a conventional presentation of cashews, PickNIC
enjoyed Mrs. May's cashew crunch. We also suggest
tossing a handful of cashew nuts into a lunch salad,
tempeh stir-fry or add-hot-water features below (25-30).

24. Oat cereal

Add water or a small box of almond milk to a cup of oat-
based cereal. Our favorite is the goji-cacao flavor by
Vigilant Eats. Umpqua Oats are delicious and fairly
priced, however we found some flavors to be higher in
sugar than we would prefer.

25. Pad Thai (Backpackers Pantry)

There's an interesting phenomenon with the add-hot-water meals. They bring together three eclectic groups – those who want to enjoy nature, those preparing for nature to end, and those integrating natural foods into a health plan. Most PickNIC favorites are marketed to outdoor enthusiasts. Recommendations 25-30 are our top picks. Each requires adding hot water, usually to the food in the packaging.

26. Chicken teriyaki with rice (Mountain House)

27. Organic couscous and lentil curry (Wilderness Dining)

28. Organic spinach putanesca (Backpackers Pantry)

29. Split pea and carrot soup

30. Black bean and lime soup (Dr. McDougall's)

10 Beverage bests

1. Water – variations on best

Water is the best hydration. After all, beyond infancy, it's the one for which the human body was designed. Research of all kinds makes the same conclusion. We don't drink enough. So here are some new ways to fill the tank:

- Pick a glass or stainless steel water bottle with a practical cap

- Make a carrying strap for your water bottle.

- Add a dash of sea salt to filtered water.

- Add a squeeze of fresh lime juice.

- To aid digestion add a splash of red wine vinegar or apple cider vinegar.

- Download an "app" for locating water fountains.

2. Herb tea with honey

The cold weather this winter had PickNIC taste testers wishing for warm beverages. Herb teas have so many varieties we didn't select a favorite. Those who would avail themselves of lunchtime herb tea if it were a bit sweeter may wish to add honey.

Honey has been recognized since ancient times for its healing properties, and ongoing research is add to the list of health benefits. The antioxidants often credited with honey's salutary effects are derived from plants with bees as the harvesters.

The blackberry blossom honey stick and honey with added vanilla bean distributed by Bee Healthy Farms are especially flavorful and can be purchased from BeeHealthyFarms.com.

3. Electrolyte packets - Flavrz Sports and Flavrz Immunity

Bravisimo! These organic beverage packets are marketplace champions. Flavrz offers two sports beverages that are delicious and have crowd appeal. The packaging is trendy and encourages safe use of reusable water bottles. The excellent ingredients are on each packet, not just the box. We were impressed with the customer service.

When PickNIC considers short-term health impact, Flavrz comes out ahead cost-wise. For example, Flavrz ingredients can reasonably be expected to support the body following sports-related dips in immune function. And one less cold during track season would make Flavrz a bargain.

For product questions contact Valli Baker at Flavrz Organic Beverages LLC valli@flavrzorganics.com.

Flavrz Organic Drink mixes can be purchased online at www.flavrzdrinkmix.com and Amazon.

4. Hot cocoa in a small thermos

Portion size is important here and so is leveraging spices over sugar. Our first choice is made by Mars Company under the brand American Heritage Chocolate. It is a tasty spice blend with low sugar as prepared during colonial times. American Heritage Chocolate is sold through various nonprofit organizations dedicated to preserving our nation's old ways.

5. Coconut water or coconut powder

Water straight from the green coconut is best. For most of us that's not practical even if it could fit in a brown lunch bag. Any coconut beverage short of fresh has to balance food safety with minimal processing and packaging that doesn't introduce toxicants. Therefore, rather than any one brand in this quickly growing market, I would prioritize glass bottles with sealed lids.

Coconut is also available as a powder which can be reconstituted as a beverage. Coco Hydro is one such product manufactured by Big Tree Farms.

6. Cultured milk

Once children are school-aged their dairy beverages should be cultured. We suggest the same criteria for cultured milk as for yogurt – low sugar, no artificial sweeteners, and live active cultures. Cultured milk from goats or sheep is preferred. No milk product should be ultra-pasteurized since this is incompatible with sustaining live active cultures.

"Cultured" milk might well be considered an entendre since filmjólk is from Sweden, lassi from India, kefir from Russia, and so on. Each culture has its own.

7. Boxed or bottled juices

The selection of single serving containers of no-added-sugar juices is fairly small. This is probably due to the price point. PickNIC suggests diluting juices into a water bottle washed daily.

For times when the single serving is important consider R.W. Knudsen brand organic pear juice from concentrate (boxes), grapefruit (glass bottles) and organic just tart cherry (glass bottles).

8. If-you-like-it-you-need-it beverages

A recent study show that on most days most U.S. children arrive to school mildly dehydrated. What a fabulous opportunity for change! The study matches my clinical observations that approximately ¼ of youth find a thermos of warm low-sodium chicken broth tasty. Many try unflavored Pedialyte calling it "Not bad tasting." This is their body communicating a message for better hydration.

9. Greens drink

Green Vibrance by Vibrant Health single serving packets are not messy and just require emptying the packet into a water bottle. Our team found them tasty and taking needed food safety precautions.

Some beverage powders which looked initially promising are sold through vitamin companies and have little if any kid-appeal. Some organic fruit pure beverages are sold through pyramid marketing schemes, which turned us off for many reasons including food safety concerns and the inaccessibility of corporate leadership.

10. Something totally new

Try a beverage with a textured surprise. Mamma Chia's vitality beverage with the tag line "seed your soul" is an aptly named bottle of hydrated chia seeds. The blackberry hibiscus flavor looks like liquid jam. The ingredients are nutritious although sweeter than we'd prefer. The cost is higher than other beverages, but may well be worth the extra for the novelty.

We also like the health benefits of a brand of turmeric beverages sold in the U.S. by Turmeric Alive, Inc. I recommend the flavor called Vegan Elixir. The confusing thing is that the brand is spelled like turmeric but without the "r".

10 Best brown bag lunch desserts

1. Prime Number Fruit Parfait, presented by Math Tree, Inc.

Enjoy 1 cup of yogurt or low-sugar whipped cream. Add 2 slices of banana, 3 strawberries, 5 pitted cherries, 7 blueberries and then get really creative with 11 pomegranate seeds. Whichever you choose, have fun with math and making dessert. Don't be divided. Let the benefits add up.

2. Dates (pitted) with cream cheese

This long-time international tradition is one to remember. It can be quickly assembled as a lunchtime party tray.

3. Round your meal with a square of chocolate

Where the expression "square meal" originated seems mysterious. Instead of weighing in on the possible origins, I'm suggesting a new one! How about a meal topped off with 4 squares of the most delicious and nutritious chocolate you can imagine.

Salazon chocolate offers a high quality organic chocolate flavored with sea salt and cracked black pepper. The bars are gluten-free, vegan and Kosher. This is

PickNIC's favorite chocolate bar and it is currently being used in a food-related youth engagement program.

Salazon chocolate is becoming more widely available. It can be purchased at local natural food stores, Wegmans and Whole Foods. Online purchases can be placed on the following website:
www.salazonchoc.com/collections/chocolate

Spices have traditionally been added to chocolate. The classic example is mole, a Mexican chili pepper and chocolate spice blend. I interviewed anthropologist Dr. Linda Perry who shared an interesting hypothesis. Spices help conduct nerve messages from the tongue to the brain. In that way the role of salt and pepper naturally enhances the food's taste. With less sugar, I note.

4. Nuts: Glazed and chocolate-coated

Robust science proves that eating nuts is one of the best health investments we can make. Add some organic sweeteners and nuts become a dessert.

PickNIC's glazed nut pick is Sahale Snacks' Cashews with Pomegranate + Vanilla. PickNIC found the 1.5 ounce single serving packages convenient for brown bags. These can be purchased at Sahalesnacks.com under Grab & Go Snacks.

Next Organics dark chocolate Brazil nuts enhance the taste of this especially nutritious nut. Plus their natural chocolate-covered shape resembles Easter eggs.

5. Chewing gum

Medical research backs our suggestion to, "Chew in good health." Two ingredients, xylitol and propolis confer benefits which we elaborate below.

Xylichew gum was developed in Finland many years ago. Xylitol is traditionally derived from the sap of birch trees. It could be compared to maple syrup from red maple trees.

Not only is Xylichew sweetened with xylitol to avoid sugar and artificial sweeteners, the xylitol confers health benefits, too. Xylitol has been proven to reduce risk of dental cavities, ear infections and skin rashes.

Now there are at least five purveyors of xylitol chewing gum, most of which PickNIC's team has sampled. Our concern is that the newer gums use xylitol which is derived from sources other than birch trees and shouldn't be assumed to confer the same health benefits. Some brands overuse xylitol which can trigger some gas and bloating. For these reasons PickNIC recommends Xylichew brand.

Propolis comes from bees and is considered an Apitherapy product. Also called bee glue, bees use propolis to repair the hive and coat the comb. Rich in plant-derived antioxidants, propolis has emerging roles in cancer prevention and respiratory health.

The propolis-containing chewing gum we tasted is Propolia brand. We like the mint & licorice and cinnamon flavors. And we also noted that this gum is sweetened with xylitol. Made in France Propolia can be purchased from U.S. based BeeHealthyFarms.com.

6. Mints and gum drops

Kaol mints from Japan give flavor and nutrients but not calories. The intense mint flavor isn't for everyone, but those who find it a satisfying conclusion to a meal are encouraged to enjoy them.

Another acquired taste that is well worth sampling is Propolia brand gum drops. Ingredients include honey and propolis. Propolis is an Apitherapy product with health benefits described in the chewing gum entry above. Our favorite flavor is vanilla. Made in France they are called Gommes de Propolis and can be purchased from U.S. based BeeHealthyFarms.com

7. "Pudding" kids in the kitchen

Among the world's most popular and nutritious desserts is pudding. PickNIC's top examples are Peruvian purple corn pudding called mazamorra morada and Indian rice pudding with cardamom. When prepared locally and made fresh, they are delicious and nutritious. However the packaged puddings are over-sugared and only resemble the real thing. What we have found is there are plenty of reduced sugar recipes and that desserts- no matter where they are from - appeal to young kitchen helpers. Have fun "pudding" kids in the kitchen!

8. Good fortune cookies

Healthful fortunes (fortune cookies) can be made at home. One such recipe can be found at dessertswithbenefits.com/healthy-homemade-fortune-cookies.

9. "Contain" your surprise

Fox Run makes a cupcake container shaped like an ice cream cup with a clear plastic swirly lid which resembles smooth serve ice cream. PickNIC suggests using these for everything but cupcakes. Consider using this container for berries topped with low-sugar whipped cream, chocolate-coated nuts and homemade muffins when appearance matters.

Two downsides are the container's price and that it isn't dishwasher safe. We still think the presentation of food that this container provides is worth the investment.

10. Dr. Porter's Halvah Dessert

Ingredients:

2 cups (16 oz)	raw tahini (thickest consistency available)
1 ½ to 2 cups	Chatfield's natural carob chips, beet sweetened (or vegan chocolate chips)
1 tsp.	vanilla extract, alcohol free
1/4 to 1 tsp.	cinnamon powder
1 pinch	cardamom powder
1/2 to 1 cup	salted pumpkin seeds, chopped
3 Tbsp.	maple syrup (optional)

Preparation:

1. Melt the carob chips in a double boiler.

2. Combine remaining ingredients in a small mixing bowl. Stir in the nuts/seed, then pour in the melted carob and give a final stir.

3. Pour mix into an 8X8 pan and refrigerate. The mix will harden enough to cut into pieces, best to keep it cold for it will become soft if left at room temperature too long.

To purchase a healthful halvah consider Mom's Organic Munchies On-The-Go real food bar, goji and pistachio flavor. These are stored refrigerated and found in the refrigerated section of the grocery store.

Send us your favorites!
Your feedback will be helpful for PickNIC 2015. Help expand our pan-cultural menu. Perhaps one of next year's entries will be yours! Send correspondence to Ingrid@INGRIDients.com with PickNIC on the subject line.

www.ingramcontent.com/pod-product-compliance
Lightning Source LLC
Chambersburg PA
CBHW071343290326
41933CB00040B/2166